INTEGRATIVE PEDIATRICS

A Complete Guide For Nurturing Young Bodies And Harmonizing Health For Empowering Parents And Healing Children

WALTER ZYAIRE

DISCLAIMER

The information in this book is intended only for general informational purposes; it should not be used in lieu of professional advice or medical care. Since the author is not licensed to practice therapy, the information offered should not be used in place of the expertise, judgment, or guidance of qualified mental health or medical professionals. Readers are encouraged to consult therapists, medical specialists, or other qualified authorities regarding their particular situation and needs. The publisher and author disclaim all liability for any actions or decisions taken by readers based on the information in this book. Results may vary from person to person and this book's approaches, procedures, and strategies may not be suitable in all circumstances. Considering unique situations and consulting a qualified expert are essential when choosing the right course of action. Neither the publisher nor the author recommend or guarantee the efficacy of any therapy or treatment that is indicated in this book. Because the information is based on the author's research and understanding at the time of publishing, it could not reflect the most recent developments or practices in the treatment area. The publisher and the author both disclaim all liability for the accuracy, completeness, or use of the material in this book. Readers bear full responsibility for the decisions and actions they choose in light of the information presented in this book.

TABLE OF CONTENTS

CHAPTER ONE 13

OVERVIEW OF INTEGRATIVE PEDIATRICS 13

INTEGRATIVE PEDIATRICS OVERVIEW 13

THE VALUE OF INTEGRATED METHODS IN PEDIATRIC.....14

CHAPTER TWO 17

INTEGRATIVE PEDIATRICS: THE BASICS 17

INTEGRATIVE PEDIATRICS' DEFINITION AND GUIDING PRINCIPLES...17

HISTORICAL ANGLE...18

INTEGRATIVE MEDICINE'S PLACE IN PAEDIATRIC HEALTHCARE 18

EVIDENCE-BASED APPROACHES 19

CHAPTER THREE 21

COMPREHENSIVE EVALUATION AND PROGNOSIS 21

COMPREHENSIVE PEDIATRIC EVALUATION 21

INVESTIGATIVE INSTRUMENTS IN INTEGRATIVE PEDIATRICS 22

COMBINING CONVENTIONAL AND NON-TRADITIONAL APPROACHES

....22

CASE STUDIES...23

CHAPTER FOUR 25

DIETARY AND NUTRITIONAL APPROACHES.....................25

NUTRITION'S SIGNIFICANCE IN PEDIATRIC HEALTH 25

COMPREHENSIVE NUTRITIONAL GUIDELINES FOR KIDS 25

SUPPLEMENTAL NUTRITION IN PEDIATRIC CARE............26

DIETARY SPECIALISATIONS AND THEIR EFFECTS 27

CHAPTER FIVE...29

PEDIATRIC MIND-BODY MEDICINE..............................29

THE MIND-BODY LINK IN PEDIATRIC HEALTH 29

STRATEGIES FOR CHILDREN TO REDUCE STRESS.............................30

INTEGRATIVE METHODS FOR TREATING MENTAL HEALTH IN 30

FAMILY-FRIENDLY MINDFULNESS AND RELAXATION PRACTICES 31

CHAPTER SIX...33

HERBAL TREATMENTS FOR COMMON CHILDHOOD ILLNESSES 33

HERBAL MEDICINE AND NATUROPATHY IN PAEDIATRICS 33

NATURAL THERAPIES FOR CHILDREN'S HEALTH 34

INCLUDING CONVENTIONAL HEALING METHODS 35

GUIDELINES AND SAFETY 36

CHAPTER SEVEN 37

COMBINING CONVENTIONAL AND TRADITIONAL MEDICAL PRACTICES37

METHODS OF COLLABORATIVE CARE..37

COORDINATING CARE WITH PEDIATRIC SPECIALISTS 38

PROBLEMS AND SOLUTIONS IN INTEGRATIVE CARE...........................38

CASE STUDIES THAT SHOW COOPERATION 40

CHAPTER EIGHT...41

PEDIATRIC INTEGRATION IN SPECIAL POPULATIONS 41

NEONATES AND INFANTS RECEIVING INTEGRATIVE CARE.................41

PEDIATRICS FOR CHILDREN WITH CHRONIC DISEASES 42

INTEGRATIVE METHODS FOR TREATING CHILD DISABILITY 43

CULTURAL ASPECTS OF PAEDIATRIC CARE MUST BE 44

CHAPTER NINE 45

UPCOMING DEVELOPMENTS AND TRENDS 45

EMERGING TECHNOLOGIES IN PEDIATRIC INTEGRATIVE MEDICINE..45

RESEARCH AND DEVELOPMENTS IN THE FIELD...................................46

DEVELOPING INTEGRATIVE PAEDIATRICS' FUTURE.............................47

ABOUT THE BOOK

The book "Integrative Pediatrics" is a thorough and invaluable tool for medical professionals and practitioners who work with children. This book aims to improve and reshape the field of pediatric medicine through an in-depth examination of integrative methods. Integrative pediatrics is notable because of its commitment to integrating alternative and holistic modalities with standard medical techniques. This approach provides a comprehensive view that can greatly improve children's health.

A concise synopsis of the topic is given in the introduction, which also highlights the importance of integrative methods in pediatric treatment. The book explores the foundations of integrative pediatrics and clarifies the ideas that support this paradigm change in the medical field.

Highlighting the development of integrative medicine and its applicability to pediatric healthcare, a historical background is provided.

Crucially, the book has a strong emphasis on evidence-based procedures, which ensures the veracity of the information offered and grounds its content in the most recent research.

Integrative pediatrics relies heavily on holistic assessment and diagnosis, which gives practitioners a strong foundation for thoroughly assessing children's health. The use of diagnostic tools and case studies augments the material's practical applicability, rendering it an invaluable resource for practitioners aiming to incorporate integrative approaches into their work.

It also highlights the crucial role that nutrition plays in pediatric health by focusing on nutrition and dietary approaches. The book acknowledges the significant influence that specialized diets and nutritional supplements can have on a child's general health, in addition to outlining integrative dietary suggestions.

Furthermore, a sophisticated awareness of the connection between children's physical and mental health is shown in the investigation of mind-body medicine in pediatric treatment. An integrated approach to mental health, stress management strategies, and mindfulness exercises for families all contribute to a comprehensive care paradigm that transcends conventional medical bounds.

A thorough discussion of naturopathy and herbal therapy gives practitioners insight into how to integrate conventional medical approaches into pediatric treatment. To guarantee that practitioners use these modalities responsibly and morally, safety precautions are highlighted.

The partnership between conventional medicine is also covered in the book, with special emphasis placed on the necessity of coordinating care with pediatric specialists. Included case examples demonstrate effective teamwork and provide useful advice on how to overcome obstacles in integrated care.

The book gains depth from its treatment of specific populations, which includes newborns, infants, children with chronic illnesses, and people with impairments. Adapting integrative techniques to varied populations is crucial, as highlighted by the importance of cultural concerns in pediatric treatment.

"Integrative Pediatrics" is a groundbreaking work that not only enlightens but also stimulates a paradigm shift in the way pediatric care is approached. It offers a thorough manual for medical practitioners who are dedicated to improving children's health by implementing integrative approaches.

CHAPTER ONE

OVERVIEW OF INTEGRATIVE PEDIATRICS

INTEGRATIVE PEDIATRICS OVERVIEW

Integrative pediatrics is a progressive, all-encompassing approach in the field of modern healthcare that blends complementary and alternative therapies with Western mainstream medicine. This paradigm recognizes the importance of treating children as complex people influenced by a multitude of interconnected circumstances, rather than just as isolated physical entities. To give pediatric patients complete and individualized care, integrative pediatrics emphasizes the integration of evidence-based conventional medicine with complementary approaches like diet, mind-body techniques, and alternative medicines.

It is impossible to overestimate the importance of integrative approaches in pediatric care given how distinct and dynamic child development is.

Since a child's physical, emotional, and social well-being are all intertwined, integrative pediatrics goes deeper than traditional medical models, which frequently concentrate on symptom management. This method creates a more thorough and patient-centered healthcare paradigm by customizing interventions to address both the underlying causes and the symptoms.

THE VALUE OF INTEGRATED METHODS IN PEDIATRIC HEALTHCARE

Integrative pediatrics places a high value on preventive treatment, which is one of its key features. Integrative practitioners emphasize preventative approaches over-reactive treatment, equipping parents and other carers with the knowledge and resources they need to support children's general health and wellbeing. This proactive approach builds a foundation for resilience and long-term well-being in addition to improving the child's current health.

Moreover, the collaboration between medical professionals, patients, and their families is highly valued in integrative pediatrics. By actively including parents and other carers in the decision-making process, practitioners in this collaborative model acknowledge and value their important role in a child's healthcare journey. By fostering a sense of trust, improving communication, and advancing a more comprehensive understanding of the child's health, this shared responsibility makes sure that treatment plans are in line with the family's preferences and values.

 A vast range of therapeutic modalities is also included in integrative pediatrics, from traditional drugs and procedures to alternative therapies like acupuncture, chiropractic adjustments, and herbal remedies. A customized and adaptable treatment plan that takes into account the unique requirements and preferences of every child and family is made possible by this integrated approach. Practitioners seek to maximize health outcomes while reducing the possibility of therapy's adverse effects by combining the best aspects of both worlds.

Integrative Pediatrics is a paradigm change in pediatric healthcare that combines the best aspects of complementary and conventional medicine while recognizing the interconnectedness of a child's health. This strategy is significant because it can offer collaborative, preventive, and individualized care, which will eventually support pediatric patients' long-term health and holistic development. Integrative pediatrics presents a viable path forward for raising the caliber and efficacy of child healthcare as the area develops.

CHAPTER TWO

INTEGRATIVE PEDIATRICS: THE BASICS

INTEGRATIVE PEDIATRICS' DEFINITION AND GUIDING PRINCIPLES

Integrative pediatrics is a comprehensive approach to child health care that blends complementary and alternative therapies with traditional medical procedures. It places a strong emphasis on a patient-centered approach, acknowledging the value of treating medical symptoms as well as taking into account a child's emotional, social, and environmental needs. Integrative pediatrics' guiding concepts include encouraging a cooperative and understanding interaction between parents, patients, and healthcare professionals.

This method promotes general health and prevention in addition to disease care by acknowledging the individuality of every kid and customizing treatment programs accordingly.

HISTORICAL ANGLE

Integrative pediatrics has its origins in traditional medical practices that embrace a holistic view of the body and mind. Different cultures have evolved to incorporate nutritional therapies, acupuncture, and herbal medicine into their approaches to pediatric care. Integrative pediatrics rose to prominence in the contemporary era in reaction to the shortcomings of traditional treatment and the increasing need for complementary therapies. Pediatric integrative healthcare models emerged as a result of the recognition of the interdependence of health and the need for a more thorough approach.

INTEGRATIVE MEDICINE'S PLACE IN PAEDIATRIC HEALTHCARE

Integrative medicine is essential to pediatric healthcare because it broadens the range of available treatments and encourages a more individualized approach to children's health.

It emphasizes preventive measures and lifestyle changes and supports evidence-based alternative therapies in addition to mainstream medical methods. In addition to treating diseases, integrated medicine actively promotes health optimization, addresses underlying causes, and reduces treatment adverse effects in pediatrics. It aims to improve pediatric patients' general health and resilience by combining the best elements of complementary and conventional therapies.

EVIDENCE-BASED APPROACHES

To guarantee the security and effectiveness of interventions, evidence-based techniques are highly valued in integrative pediatrics. The complementary therapy field constantly searches for and incorporates scientific data to support its approaches, even though some may not have undergone thorough clinical trials. This evidence-based method entails a thorough assessment of complementary and alternative medicine, dietary supplements, and mind-body techniques. Integrative pediatric practitioners make sure that the integration of complementary therapies is based on a strong scientific foundation by giving priority to beneficial interventions. The dedication to evidence-based practices upholds Integrative Pediatrics' legitimacy in the eyes of the larger medical community and advances the continuous advancement of pediatric healthcare.

CHAPTER THREE

COMPREHENSIVE EVALUATION AND PROGNOSIS

COMPREHENSIVE PEDIATRIC EVALUATION

In pediatric treatment, holistic assessment emphasizes a thorough method that takes into account a child's physical, emotional, social, and environmental well-being, among other dimensions. Integrative pediatric assessment is a key component of this strategy, which combines traditional medical examinations with complementary and alternative techniques to present a comprehensive picture of a child's health.

This holistic viewpoint acknowledges the interdependence of many facets of a child's life and health as well as the influence of diverse elements on general well-being.

INVESTIGATIVE INSTRUMENTS IN INTEGRATIVE PEDIATRICS

Integrative pediatrics uses a variety of diagnostic methods, including both standard and non-conventional examinations. To discover and diagnose medical diseases, conventional methods may include physical examinations, laboratory testing, and imaging studies. However, Integrative Pediatrics incorporates non-traditional tools including mind-body therapies, nutritional assessments, and biofeedback, going beyond the conventional approaches. These resources aid medical practitioners in comprehending a child's health on a deeper level by taking into account not only the physical symptoms but also the emotional and environmental factors.

COMBINING CONVENTIONAL AND NON-TRADITIONAL APPROACHES

A cornerstone of holistic assessment and diagnosis is the integration of conventional and non-conventional techniques. While alternative approaches include a wide range of techniques like herbal medicine, acupuncture, and mind-body treatments, traditional approaches frequently contain evidence-based procedures with roots in Western medicine. Integrative pediatrics seeks to close the gap between these methods, appreciating their respective contributions to comprehensive evaluation and individual child care. To provide thorough and individualized care, this inclusive approach encourages collaboration among healthcare specialists from diverse disciplines.

CASE STUDIES

Case studies are essential for showing how Integrative Pediatric Assessment and Diagnosis is used in real-world situations. These real-world instances shed light on how medical practitioners combine conventional and non-conventional techniques to manage the intricacies of a child's health. Case examples highlight the combination of several diagnostic instruments, the cooperation of many medical professionals, and the customized strategy to meet the unique requirements of every kid. The examination of case studies facilitates a more profound comprehension of the obstacles and achievements encountered while introducing an integrative approach in pediatric healthcare, hence aiding in the continuous advancement of optimal practices within the domain.

Integrative Pediatric Assessment and Diagnosis provides a complete framework for assessing and treating a child's health by integrating conventional and unconventional techniques. Healthcare practitioners can improve their capacity to deliver individualized and successful care for pediatric patients by utilizing a variety of diagnostic techniques and reviewing real-world case studies. This is because pediatric patients have complex interactions between physical, emotional, social, and environmental aspects.

CHAPTER FOUR

DIETARY AND NUTRITIONAL APPROACHES

NUTRITION'S SIGNIFICANCE IN PEDIATRIC HEALTH

Since nutrition is a major factor in a child's growth, development, and general well-being, it is important for pediatric health. Sustaining childhood development's rapid physical and cognitive growth requires adequate nourishment. Beyond just providing for bodily needs, nutrition has a critical role in the development of healthy tissues, organs, and immune systems in children. Diets high in nutrients help reduce the risk of nutritional deficiencies and lay the groundwork for a healthy lifestyle that continues into adulthood.

COMPREHENSIVE NUTRITIONAL GUIDELINES FOR KIDS

The goal of integrated dietary guidelines for kids is to offer all-encompassing advice that takes into account the various nutritional requirements at various growth stages. The significance of a balanced diet that includes a range of dietary groups, such as fruits, vegetables, whole grains, lean proteins, and dairy products, is emphasized by these guidelines. Promoting healthful eating practices at an early age helps children develop a positive relationship with food and lays the groundwork for long-term well-being. To encourage healthy eating habits, integrative approaches also emphasize the value of family engagement, education, and the establishment of a supportive environment.

SUPPLEMENTAL NUTRITION IN PEDIATRIC CARE

Nutritional supplements are occasionally advised in pediatric care to support certain medical conditions or treat particular deficiencies. Supplements can be helpful in situations where dietary consumption may be inadequate or when there are increased nutritional requirements owing to illness, growth spurts, or other circumstances, even though a well-balanced diet should ideally offer all the necessary elements. Vitamins, minerals, and omega-3 fatty acids are common supplements; each has a unique function in supporting a child's health, from bone formation to cognitive function.

DIETARY SPECIALISATIONS AND THEIR EFFECTS

Pediatric health can be significantly impacted by specialized diets made to fit particular dietary requirements or medical problems. For instance, children with certain medical disorders like celiac disease, lactose intolerance, or epilepsy may benefit from diets like gluten-free, dairy-free, or ketogenic diets. To make sure that any special diet fits the child's nutritional needs and does not negatively impact their general health, carers and medical professionals must collaborate. To create and keep track of these customized nutrition regimens, a multidisciplinary approach comprising pediatricians, dietitians, and other specialists are frequently required.

Nutrition plays a critical role in a child's growth, development, and general health. Integrative dietary guidelines emphasize balanced and diverse diets and support a comprehensive approach to child nutrition. In certain situations, nutritional supplements could be advised, and certain diets might be helpful in the management of particular medical disorders. In the end, encouraging children to eat healthily lays the groundwork for a lifetime of well-being, therefore thoughtful consideration of nutritional strategies is essential in pediatric treatment.

CHAPTER FIVE

PEDIATRIC MIND-BODY MEDICINE

THE MIND-BODY LINK IN PEDIATRIC HEALTH

The mind-body link, which highlights the complex interactions between children's psychological and physical health, is important for pediatric health. Acknowledging this relationship is crucial to comprehending and managing a range of health concerns.

According to research, a child's mental and emotional well-being can have a big impact on their physical health, affecting things like immunological response, hormone balance, and general resilience. In pediatrics, fostering a positive mind-body link includes advancing mental health in general, stress reduction, and emotional well-being.

STRATEGIES FOR CHILDREN TO REDUCE STRESS

It is essential to use stress reduction strategies specifically designed for kids to lessen the damaging effects of stress on their growing bodies and minds. Stressors can take many different shapes for kids, from social difficulties to scholastic obligations. Age-appropriate methods of reducing stress, such as guided visualization, deep breathing exercises, and art or play therapy, are all included in mind-body medicine for pediatric patients. These methods seek to provide kids with coping skills so they can better handle stress and develop resilience.

INTEGRATIVE METHODS FOR TREATING MENTAL HEALTH IN CHILDREN

The efficacy of integrative approaches—which blend traditional medical interventions with complementary and alternative therapies—in the field of pediatric mental health is becoming increasingly acknowledged.

Pediatric integrative medicine places a strong emphasis on a comprehensive view of the patient's health, taking into account not just the physical symptoms but also the emotional, social, and environmental aspects that can affect mental health. Children who are experiencing mental health issues can receive comprehensive care through the work of medical specialists, mental health practitioners, and complementary therapies.

FAMILY-FRIENDLY MINDFULNESS AND RELAXATION PRACTICES

The benefits of mindfulness and relaxation methods for enhancing family well-being are becoming more widely acknowledged. Families are essential to a child's growth and development, and the mental health of the family as a whole can have a big impact on the child's general well-being. Introducing mindfulness exercises to families promotes a common feeling of emotional equilibrium and relaxation. Family-focused practices like mindful eating, meditation, and relaxation exercises help improve the environment for a child's mental and emotional development while also strengthening the relationships within the family.

Pediatric mind-body medicine emphasizes the complex relationship between children's physical and mental health. Healthcare providers can support children's holistic well-being by embracing integrative approaches to pediatric mental health, teaching mindfulness and relaxation practices within the family, and incorporating stress reduction measures. Building a strong mind-body bond at a young age lays the groundwork for lifelong resilience and good health.

CHAPTER SIX
HERBAL TREATMENTS FOR COMMON CHILDHOOD ILLNESSES

HERBAL MEDICINE AND NATUROPATHY IN PAEDIATRICS

Throughout history, herbal medicine has played a significant role in healthcare, and its potential efficacy and safety in pediatrics are beginning to be recognized. Herbs are used to treat common pediatric illnesses, providing a natural substitute for prescription drugs. For example, chamomile and ginger are frequently used to treat digestive problems in newborns, such as colic and indigestion. Due to their immune-boosting qualities, Echinacea and elderberry may be taken into consideration for the treatment of recurrent infections in children, such as the flu and colds. Herbal medicines are especially popular because of their mild character, which offers a comprehensive approach to supporting a child's entire well-being in pediatric conditions.

Naturopathy seeks to locate and treat the underlying causes of health issues while highlighting the body's inherent capacity for self-healing. Naturopathic methods for pediatric wellness include an emphasis on a comprehensive view of a child's health, taking into account aspects including lifestyle, diet, and mental health.

A key component of naturopathic pediatric care is dietary interventions, such as introducing foods high in nutrients and removing possible allergies. Furthermore, lifestyle changes—like promoting outdoor activities and getting enough sleep—are stressed as a way to improve general health and ward off frequent childhood illnesses. Naturopathic doctors collaborate with parents to design individualized strategies that promote the child's best possible growth and development.

INCLUDING CONVENTIONAL HEALING METHODS

The incorporation of conventional medical procedures into pediatric care recognizes the wide range of national healthcare systems. Ayurveda, Traditional Chinese Medicine (TCM), and Native American medicine are examples of traditional systems that provide distinctive viewpoints on health and healing. Using therapies that are in line with traditional ideas and having a thorough understanding of each child's unique constitution is necessary for integrating these traditions into pediatric care.

TCM, for instance, may include acupuncture or specially prepared herbal remedies for children. This holistic approach promotes a more thorough and patient-centered form of care by taking into accounts the child's emotional and spiritual well-being in addition to treating physical problems.

GUIDELINES AND SAFETY

It is crucial to guarantee the safety of naturopathic treatments and herbal medicine in pediatric care. Before proposing any herbal treatments or naturopathic interventions, practitioners in this discipline stress the significance of evidence-based procedures and comprehensive examinations. To avoid side effects, dosage modifications according to age, weight, and specific medical problems are essential. It is recommended that conventional healthcare providers collaborate to enable a comprehensive strategy that integrates the advantages of both modern and traditional treatment. To coordinate complete care that puts the child's safety and well-being first, parents are recommended to speak with licensed practitioners who have experience with pediatric herbal medicine and naturopathy and to have open communication with their child's primary healthcare physician.

CHAPTER SEVEN

COMBINING CONVENTIONAL AND TRADITIONAL MEDICAL PRACTICES

METHODS OF COLLABORATIVE CARE

Integrating conventional medicine requires using collaborative care strategies that put patients' overall health first. Healthcare professionals from various backgrounds, such as naturopaths, mainstream medical practitioners, and traditional healers, are brought together by this interdisciplinary approach.

The objective is to take advantage of both systems' advantages while acknowledging that each has special things to offer. Through this partnership, patients' health is better understood holistically, taking into account not only their physical symptoms but also their emotional, social, and cultural dimensions of health.

COORDINATING CARE WITH PEDIATRIC SPECIALISTS

The combination of traditional medicine becomes especially important when it comes to pediatric healthcare. A comprehensive awareness of the child's medical requirements as well as the possible advantages of sticking to conventional techniques is necessary when coordinating care with pediatric specialists. To develop a smooth and unique care plan, pediatric specialists collaborate closely with conventional practitioners and traditional healers. Through this partnership, the family's choices and values are taken into consideration while ensuring the kid receives the most effective and culturally sensitive care possible.

PROBLEMS AND SOLUTIONS IN INTEGRATIVE CARE

There are several difficulties in combining conventional treatment. The differing viewpoints and skepticism that might exist between practitioners of different medical traditions are a significant barrier. Open communication, respect for one another, and continual education to promote understanding are necessary to close this gap. Furthermore, establishing evidence-based procedures and standardizing methods contribute to the development of trust between patients and healthcare providers. Establishing mutual understanding regarding the objectives of patient welfare promotes a more seamless integration procedure.

The legal and regulatory structures that control the healthcare industry present another difficulty. Navigating the legal system can be difficult, and integrative treatment frequently operates in grey areas. It is crucial to create precise rules and regulations that recognize and encourage cooperative methods. To foster an atmosphere that supports and governs integrative treatment, legislators, healthcare facilities, and professional associations must actively participate in this.

CASE STUDIES THAT SHOW COOPERATION

Analyzing real-world case studies offers insightful information about effective cooperation between conventional medicines. These examples highlight the benefits of integrated treatments and show how well merging various healing modalities can work. A case study could demonstrate how, in the context of post-surgical treatment, acupuncture enhances traditional pain management techniques and promotes patient satisfaction and recovery. These drawings are potent demonstrations of the concrete advantages that result from medical practitioners working together and utilizing the best aspects of many medical traditions.

A dedication to collaborative care approaches is necessary for the integration of traditional and contemporary medicine, particularly in pediatric settings. Even though there are obstacles, proactive measures like open dialogue, education, and the creation of laws that support them can be taken to address them.

CHAPTER EIGHT

PEDIATRIC INTEGRATION IN SPECIAL POPULATIONS

NEONATES AND INFANTS RECEIVING INTEGRATIVE CARE

This fragile population's particular needs are addressed through a comprehensive approach. Integrative pediatrics is founded on the principles of optimizing the general health of infants and young children by fusing evidence-based complementary therapies with conventional medical methods. Practitioners may use music therapy, soft touch, and massage treatment in neonatal care to encourage healthy development, lessen stress, and foster bonding.

To treat certain health issues and encourage healthy growth, nutritional interventions, such as customized meals or supplementation, may also be taken into consideration. The goal of the joint efforts of pediatricians, neonatologists, and integrative practitioners is to improve the standard of care that newborns and neonates receive.

PEDIATRICS FOR CHILDREN WITH CHRONIC DISEASES

Managing enduring health issues in children with chronic diseases requires a comprehensive and integrated approach. Integrative pediatricians work in conjunction with other medical professionals and therapists to provide individualized treatment programs that include complementary therapies, lifestyle changes, and traditional medical approaches. Children suffering from long-term health issues like diabetes or asthma, for instance, could find relief from a combination of medical interventions and complementary therapies like acupuncture, breathing techniques, or dietary changes. Enhancing symptom management, raising the child's quality of life, and enabling families to take an active role in their child's care are the objectives.

INTEGRATIVE METHODS FOR TREATING CHILD DISABILITY

Integrative approaches to pediatric disabilities acknowledge the multifaceted nature of disabilities and seek to improve a child's overall well-being by addressing not only the physical but also the emotional, social, and cognitive domains. To give a comprehensive and tailored approach, complementary modalities like yoga, mindfulness, and art therapy are frequently combined with therapies like occupational therapy, physical therapy, and speech therapy.

For kids with impairments, the main goals are to maximize functional capacities, promote independence, and enhance overall quality of life. Integrative care recognizes that to provide a supportive environment for children with disabilities, teamwork between educators, families, and healthcare providers is essential.

CULTURAL ASPECTS OF PAEDIATRIC CARE MUST BE CONSIDERED

The importance of acknowledging and honoring children's varied cultural backgrounds is underscored by cultural concerns in pediatric treatment. Integrative pediatricians make an effort to comprehend the cultural background of each patient, taking into account customs, beliefs, and behaviors that could have an impact on well-being and health. Effective communication and cooperation with families from various cultural backgrounds are key components of this strategy, which guarantees that healthcare plans are sensitive to cultural differences and consistent with the family's beliefs. The effectiveness of healthcare interventions is eventually increased when cultural competence is incorporated into pediatric care, as it promotes trust and strengthens patient-doctor relationships. All pediatric patients benefit from a more inclusive and fair healthcare experience when cultural diversity is acknowledged.

CHAPTER NINE

UPCOMING DEVELOPMENTS AND TRENDS

EMERGING TECHNOLOGIES IN PEDIATRIC INTEGRATIVE MEDICINE

With the introduction of state-of-the-art technologies, Pediatric Integrative Medicine is undergoing a revolutionary phase. The use of augmented reality (AR) and virtual reality (VR) in pediatric healthcare is one noteworthy development. With the help of this immersive and interactive technology, pain management, anxiety reduction, and treatments can be achieved in novel ways. Virtual reality (VR) has demonstrated the potential to divert children during medical procedures, hence enhancing their overall healthcare experience.

Furthermore, a major factor in increasing access to pediatric integrative treatment is telemedicine. More and more follow-ups, monitoring, and consultations are being conducted remotely, particularly in places with little healthcare resources. The transition to digital health solutions promotes a more patient-centric and easily accessible healthcare system by guaranteeing prompt treatments and continuous support for pediatric patients.

RESEARCH AND DEVELOPMENTS IN THE FIELD

There have been notable advances in both clinical and research in the field of pediatric integrative medicine. To develop individualized and focused therapies, researchers are exploring the molecular and genetic foundations of a variety of pediatric illnesses. Precision medicine has the potential to improve outcomes, reduce side effects, and customize therapies for specific children.

In addition, research on mind-body therapies in pediatric healthcare is becoming more and more important. The effectiveness of mindfulness exercises, yoga, and relaxation techniques in treating chronic illnesses, lowering stress levels, and improving general well-being in pediatric patients is being researched. The incorporation of these holistic methods into traditional medical practice is a sign of a more general change in the direction of a patient-centered, all-inclusive healthcare paradigm.

DEVELOPING INTEGRATIVE PAEDIATRICS' FUTURE

A holistic approach that considers pediatric patients' emotional, mental, and social well-being in addition to their physical health is what will define integrative pediatrics in the future.

It is becoming more common for healthcare professionals—including doctors, psychiatrists, dietitians, and complementary therapists—to collaborate across multiple disciplines. This collaborative model addresses the various needs of young patients while guaranteeing a thorough and integrated approach to pediatric healthcare.

In addition, the application of machine learning (ML) and artificial intelligence (AI) in pediatric healthcare has the potential to completely transform treatment and diagnosis protocols. Large-scale datasets can be analyzed by AI algorithms, which can also spot trends and help healthcare professionals make decisions that are more timely and accurate. This improves healthcare delivery efficiency and helps create more individualized and successful treatment plans for kids with complicated medical issues.

Cutting-edge research, new technologies, and a move towards a more patient-centered and holistic approach are all contributing to the rapid evolution of pediatric integrative medicine. These developments could enhance pediatric patients' overall health and pave the way for the seamless integration of integrative care into pediatric healthcare systems across the globe in the future.